Taking Immunizations Safely

Quick Read

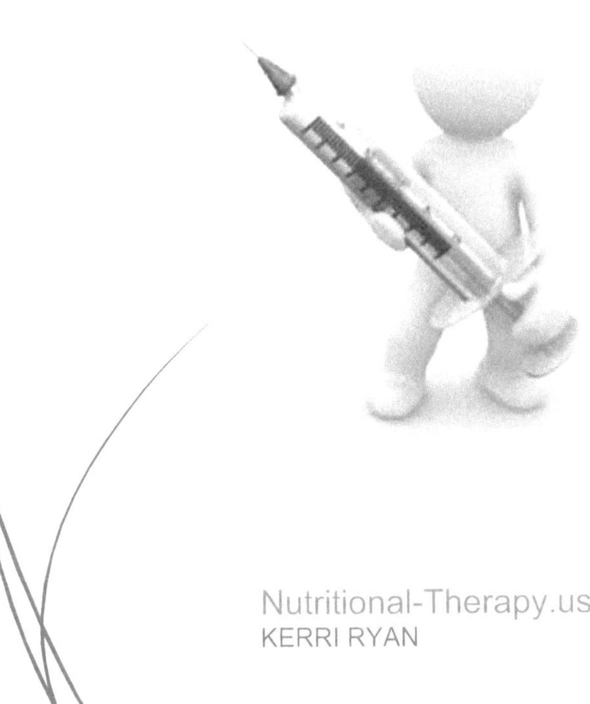

Nutritional-Therapy.us

KERRI RYAN

Taking Vaccines Safely
Quick Read

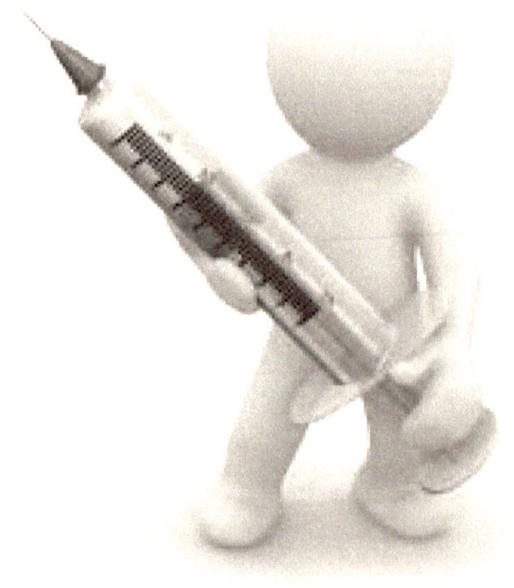

Nutritional-Therapy.us

Kerri Ryan

Contents

IMMUNIZATIONS

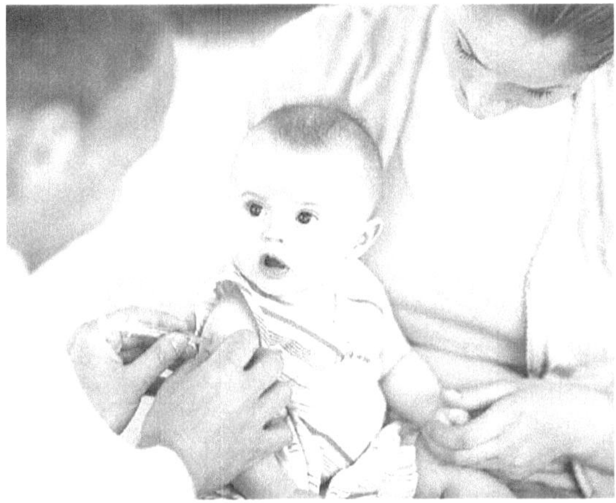

The biggest thing on everyone's mind these days is, what about the COVID-19 vaccine. Let me say from the start that while I do believe in vaccines, I do not put my faith in this one. The reason being is that this particular vaccine, in all its forms, and from all the manufacturers alter the RNA/ DNA of the recipient and will have a lasting effect, that has too many implications, to just be accepted so widely, and without proper testing. For this reason, I will make this disclaimer, and talk only about other vaccines in general, and not the COVID-19 and all its implications that are becoming known with each passing day.

We live in strange times. It is a time when we cannot enroll our kids in school unless they get immunized; yet science is now showing how some immunizations are actually harming them. How can we know what is best for our children? How can we tell if we are being told the whole truth or not? Are the effects of immunizations worth the risks involved?

Actually, both schools of thought are right. The issue is not in the immunization as much as it is in the child's ability to produce a defense against the introduction of new disease. Once we learn what immunizations are, what their purpose is, and how the body reacts to them, only then will we be able to make a sensible decision about immunizations and whether they are good for our kids.

Many Anti-Vaccine proponents believe that by allowing the government to mandate our medical care, this is putting us in a very dangerous position. Not only to becoming infected with new pathogen but causing us to lose even more of our freedoms one step at a time. If the government can decide who is 'acceptable' and who is not, they can then theoretically dictate who lives, and who dies. Giving the government this kind of control in our lives is something many people are not willing to do, and rightly so. These arguments are true to a point. However, letting our kids be subjected to known pathogens that are increasing mortality rates around the world is also not a reasonable solution.

UNFOUNDED CONCERNS

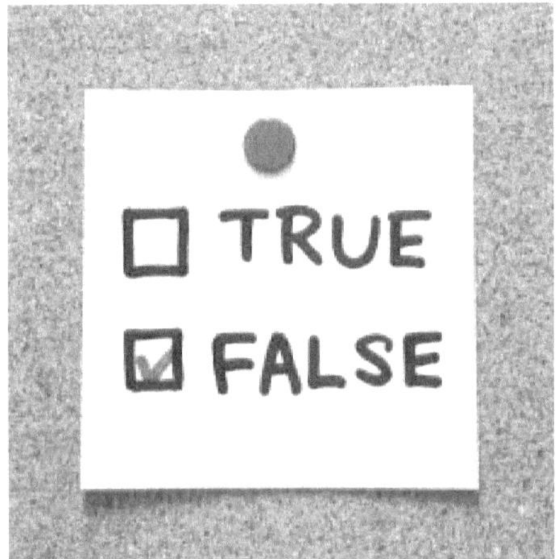

Some of the concerns people have surrounding vaccinations are for the most part unfounded. In the early days of vaccinations, around the 1950's, there were some issues, but they largely stemmed from specific manufacturers, and not the entire medical community. Over the years, vaccinations have been studied and improved, and are currently so heavily regulated that all the past concerns have been addressed and corrected. Generally speaking, the ingredients in vaccines are safe in the amounts used today.[1]

Ever hear the term 'Mad as a Hatter'? This is because back in the day, people who worked on felt hats used large amounts of Mercury to clean and protect the felt. This Mercury was absorbed through their skin, attached itself onto their nervous system, and caused them to go 'crazy'. Mercury is one of the biggest concerns among parents that are convinced it causes Autism.

Autism has many factors to it, and there is an entire spectrum of signs and symptoms, so it is not an objective claim that vaccinations alone are the cause of behaviors such as Autism. Ingredients, such as mercury, thimerosal, formaldehyde, and aluminum, can be harmful in large doses but they are not used in harmful quantities in vaccines. Children are exposed to more aluminum in breast milk and infant formula than they are exposed to in vaccines. Paul Offit, MD, notes that children are exposed to more bacteria, viruses, toxins, and other harmful substances in one day of normal activity than are in vaccines.[2] With the exception of inactivated flu vaccines, thimerosal (a mercury compound) has been removed or reduced to trace amounts in vaccines for children under 6 years old.[3] The FDA requires up to 10 or more years of testing for all vaccines before they are licensed and administered to the public, and then they are monitored by the CDC and the FDA to make sure the vaccines and the ingredients used in all vaccines are safe.[4] [56]

Except for the COVID-19 vaccine, this is the standard protocol. The COVID vaccine has bypassed all the standard protocols and was pushed through and mandated because of a 'national emergency'. It is not my belief that bypassing safety measures should ever be put aside for the greater good. The measures are put in place for the greater good, and will protect more people in the long run.

It is my opinion that some of the dangers found in vaccines are more likely due to taking too many at once or giving them to someone with an underdeveloped immune system. Injecting too many pathogens into anyone who with a compromised immune system is always a cause for concern.

By the time you have finished reading this book, you will have enough understanding to decide for yourself, what is the best course of action for you and your family before, during and after taking any vaccination. Going without them has its own cause for concern that we will look at further into this reading.

THE DIFFERENCE BETWEEN A BACTERIA AND A VIRUS

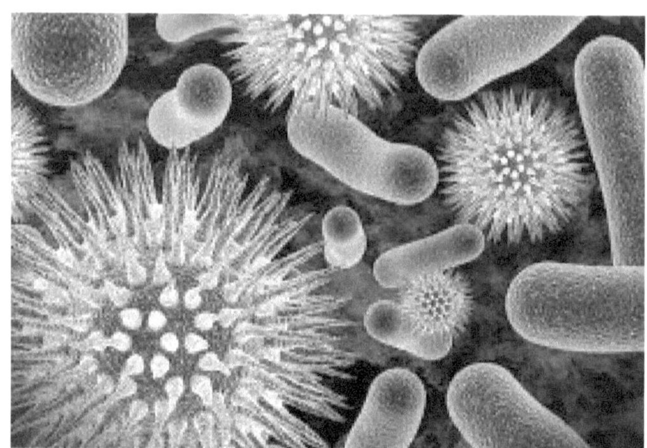

If you are going to understand bacterial and viral infections, you should start with a few basics. The main difference between a bacterium and a virus is that a bacterium can be stopped with the use of an antibiotic that kills all bacteria in the body, including the good ones we need. Therefore, doctors tell us to eat something probiotic like yogurt, along with the antibiotic, so we can replace the bacteria we need.

The issue with viruses is that we can't just take a pill and kill them, they typically need to run their course. Therefore, building a strong immune system is more important than just taking a vaccination. Without this in place, vaccines may not work. Vaccines cannot prevent a virus, but it can lessen the symptoms, and speed up recovery by exposing the body to a mild form of the pathogen, to help the body recognize it if it should ever show up in an overwhelming way.

So again, I will point out that it is always a strong immune system that stops a virus, and not the vaccine.

THE DIFFERENCE BETWEEN A VACCINE AND AN IMMUNIZATION

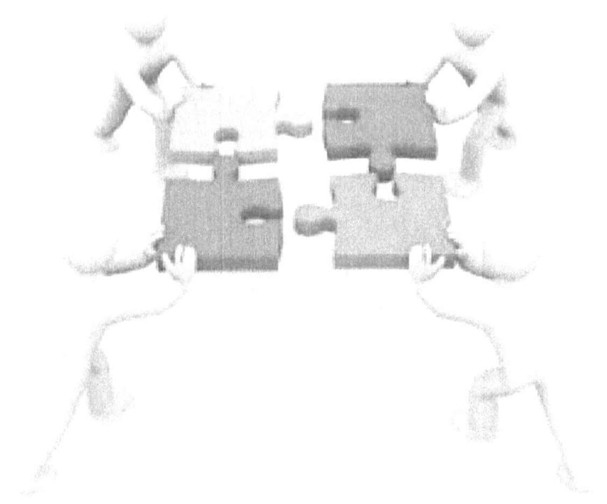

A Vaccination is when a vaccine is administered to the patient, and an Immunization is what happens in the body after they have been vaccinated. The vaccine stimulates the patient's immune system so that it can produce the proper antibodies to recognize the threat if it ever shows up in the future. It is an altered biological agent, that provides an active stimulated immunity to a specific disease. Today's vaccinations typically contain an agent that resembles a disease-causing microorganism and is often made from weakened or killed forms of the microbe, its toxins, or one of its surface proteins.

It is generally believed that vaccinations are the best way to provide protection, but this is only true if the person's immune system is strong enough to rally a defense.

Vaccines have historically been one of the main reasons why the American healthcare system has been so successful, and we should be taking some of them to provide a reasonable and rational defense. America has eradicated scores of infectious diseases that have taken millions of lives a year, all over the planet.

Below is a list of some of the diseases that the United States has successfully eradicated from our society within the last 100 years, and vaccinations that I believe should be on everyone's 'MUST HAVE' list.

THE 'MUST HAVES' OF VACCINES

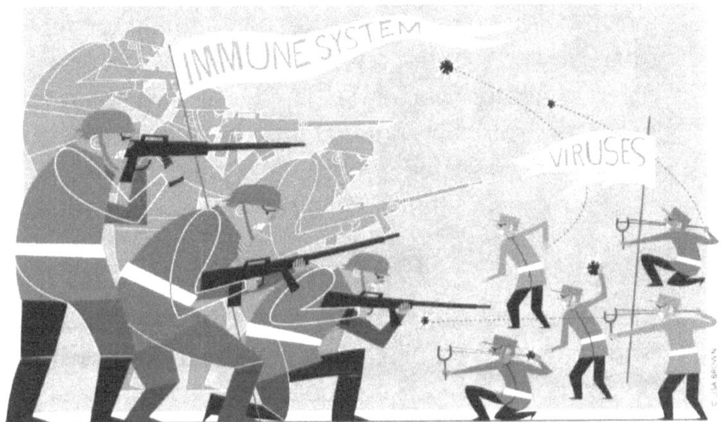

Polio

Polio is a crippling and potentially deadly infectious disease that is caused by the poliovirus. The virus spreads from person to person typically through unclean water. Once infected, the virus can invade an infected person's brain and spinal cord, causing paralysis. Polio was eliminated in the United States through a national immunization program and has for the most part kept this country polio-free. However, because of irresponsible immigration, polio is making a comeback and is becoming a threat in some parts of our country once again. The polio vaccination is definitely one that everyone should have at the recommended age.

Tetanus

Tetanus causes painful muscle stiffness and lockjaw producing results that can sometimes be fatal. Nowadays, the tetanus vaccine is part of a disease-fighting vaccine called DTaP, which provides protection against tetanus, diphtheria, and pertussis (whooping cough). Like polio, this is another vaccine that should be on the required list

Diphtheria

Most of us only know diphtheria as a vague disease from long ago, thanks to the diphtheria vaccine babies get. This vaccine, called DTaP, provides protection against diphtheria, tetanus, and pertussis (whooping cough). While preventable, diphtheria does still exist. It can cause a thick covering in the back of the nose or throat that makes it hard to breathe or swallow. Diphtheria can also lead to heart failure, paralysis, and even death. Make sure to vaccinate in order to help keep this dangerous infection away from your kids.

Pertussis- Whooping Cough

Whooping cough, or pertussis, is a highly contagious disease that can be deadly for babies. Whooping cough can cause uncontrollable, violent coughing which often makes it hard to breathe. Its "whooping" name comes from the sharp air intake sound right after a coughing fit. In babies, this disease can also cause life-threatening pauses in breathing with no cough at all. Whooping cough is especially dangerous to babies who are too young to be vaccinated themselves. Mothers should get the whooping cough vaccine during each pregnancy to pass some protection to their babies before birth. It is very important for your baby to get the whooping cough vaccine on time so he can start building his own protection against the disease.

Hepatitis A

The Hepatitis A vaccine was developed in 1995 and since then has dramatically cut the number of cases in the United States. Hepatitis A is a contagious liver disease and is transmitted through person-to-person contact or through contaminated food and water. Vaccinating against hepatitis A is a good way to help you and your family bypass Hep A for life.

Hepatitis B

Hepatitis B is spread through blood and other bodily fluids. It's especially dangerous for babies, since the hepatitis B virus can spread from an infected mother to child during birth. About nine out of every 10 infants who contract it from their mothers become permanently infected, which is why babies should get the first dose of the hepatitis B vaccine shortly after birth. Remember, the Hep B vaccine is an altered state of the virus, not a full dose that risks giving Hepatitis B to your child. All pregnant women should be tested, and all babies should be vaccinated.

Measles

People can get the measles simply by being in a room where a person with measles has been, even up to two hours after that person has left. Measles is very contagious, and it can be serious, especially for young children. There is a new trend taking place where parents are taking their kids to parties where their kids will become exposed to the measles and chickenpox, specifically so they can develop an immunity to it. This is very dangerous and should be stopped right away. The measles vaccine has been treated so that it will not infect the person, but only allow them to develop an immunity to it. Purposefully exposing anyone to a known disease is a crime and not responsible parenting. All counties in each State has free or low-cost vaccinations available, so there is really no excuse for not getting anyone vaccinated properly, and safely.

Mumps

Mumps is best known for causing puffy cheeks and a swollen jaw. This is due to swelling of the salivary glands. Other symptoms include fever, head and muscle aches, and tiredness. Mumps is a contagious disease with no real treatment, like most viruses they just need to run their course. However, there is much you can do to relieve discomfort and speed up the process. Getting the immunization is only one of the ways to combat it. Mumps is still a threat today. In recent years, mumps outbreaks have occurred in settings where there was close, extended contact with infected people, such as being in the same classroom or playing on the same sports team. The MMR vaccine protects you and your family against mumps, measles, and rubella, and is highly recommended.

Rubella

Rubella is spread by coughing and sneezing. It is especially dangerous for a pregnant woman and her developing baby. If an unvaccinated pregnant woman gets infected with rubella, she can have a miscarriage, or her baby could die shortly after birth. Also, she can pass the disease to her developing baby who can develop serious birth defects. Make sure you and your children are protected from rubella by getting vaccinated on schedule.

HIB

HIB (or its official name, Hemophilus influenzae type B) isn't as well-known as some of the other diseases, thanks to vaccines. HIB can do some serious damage to our children's immune systems and cause brain damage, hearing loss, or even death. HIB mostly affects kids under five years old. Thankfully, because of vaccinations, this has become one of the infections that has largely been eradicated in the US.

Pneumonia

This disease is caused by bacteria called Streptococcus pneumoniae. It causes ear infections, sinus infections, pneumonia, and even meningitis, making it very dangerous for children. The germs can invade parts of the body such as the brain or spinal cord, that are normally free from germs. This is also a highly recommended vaccination that will help make sure you keep kids safe from this dangerous disease.

Influenza

Flu is a respiratory illness caused by the influenza virus that infects the nose, throat, and lungs. Influenza can affect people differently based on their immune system, age, and health. Flu symptoms in children can include coughing, fever, aches, fatigue, vomiting, and diarrhea. Dehydration can be one of the biggest threats to any disease as it leaves the person less able to implement a health building response since whatever medicine goes in, comes right back out. The best way to protect babies against flu is for the mother to get a flu vaccine during pregnancy and for all caregivers and close contacts of the infant to be vaccinated. The Center for Disease Control (CDC) recommends that Everyone 6 months and older should get a flu vaccine every year. On the other hand, the flu vaccine is not mandatory, so supporting the immune system and making sure it is strong is the best way to avoid any kind of infection.

Rotavirus

Rotavirus is contagious and can cause severe watery diarrhea, often with vomiting, fever, and abdominal pain, mostly in infants and young children. In some cases, children can become severely dehydrated from the disease and need to be hospitalized. If a dehydrated child does not get needed care, they could die. The Rotavirus is another recommended vaccination that infants should receive early in life.

Chickenpox

Chickenpox is a disease that causes an itchy rash of blisters and a fever. A person with chickenpox may have as many as 500 blisters all over their body once infected. Chickenpox can be serious and even life-threatening, especially in babies, adults, and people with weakened immune systems. Even healthy children can get sick Vaccinating kids at an early age is especially important to protect your children from this fairly common disease.[7]

This list of vaccinations is one that I personally recommend for all people, at their recommended ages. There are more vaccinations available, but I am not aware of how effective they are, nor do I believe that they will bring any added protection. My approach to bacteria and viruses is to take the mandatory vaccinations, and at the same time make the body's immune system stronger, so that it can defend itself no matter what comes its way. Bacteria and viruses are living organisms that evolve to overcome vaccinations and antibiotics by mutating. By Making the body's immune system stronger, this will allow it to defend itself no matter what comes its way. This seems to be a more complete reaction instead of chasing after a mutating force that changes with each passing year.

DEVELOPING A HEALTHY IMMUNE SYSTEM

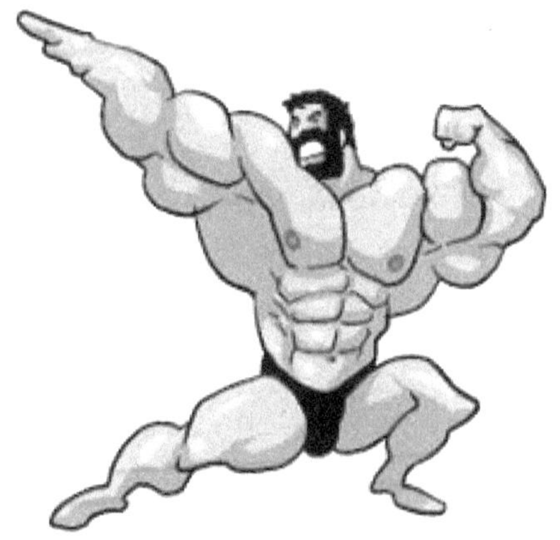

There is no 'one thing' that will make a person strong and healthy, because there are a few things that need to come together, to produce the best result. To understand exactly what happens physiologically during an infection, on a cellular level, sign up for my emails on my web site at www.Nutritional-Therapy.us and get a free eBook on ***How To Stop Infections Before They Start***. This book focuses on how bacteria and virus' respond at a cellular level, for those of you who want to know more detail about what is going on at a time like this.

The law prevents me from using words like 'treat', 'cure', 'heal;' or even imply that any supplements can be used in place of a licensed doctor, and this is true to some degree. If supplements are not improving your condition, go to a doctor, get a checkup, and make sure there are no other circumstances at play. Once again, this eBook is written to provide support to your medical doctors' advice and help to improve your child's overall defense against any immunizations they might be getting. When it comes to immunizations, I do recommend them highly, and suggest that by adding specific nutrition along with them, they can be taken safely, effectively, and without concern.

VITAMIN C

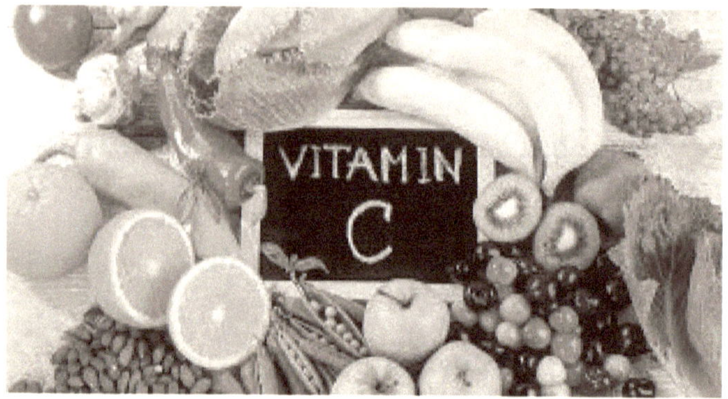

It sounds so cliché, but what is it about Vitamin C that makes it so good to the inner workings of the human body? Truthfully, this should be the first supplement to take when concerns about immunizations, bacteria or viruses are present. Multiple protective functions take place when we start taking Vitamin C at the first sign of sickness.

> It improves adrenal function that starts the whole immune system process.[8]
> It stimulates the production of antibodies[9]
> It increases the number of white cells,[10] as well as their ability to destroy bacteria[11]

A normal white cell count is typically 5000 white cells per microliter (4.5 to 11.0 × 109/L). A higher count means an infection is present and the body is fighting it. A lower count means the body is losing the battle. When as little as 1000 mg of Vitamin C are taken hourly during a cold, the white cell count immediately starts to go up to 9000 109/L or more within the day.[12] The individual and their illness will dictate how much vitamin C should be taken, but since it is not toxic, there is little concern about taking too much. Any excess is just spilled out into the urine and removed from the body.

Some of the signs and symptoms of a Vitamin C deficiency will include,[13]

> Hangnails
> Bruising
> Bleeding gums
> Nose bleeds
> Hemorrhages

The reason behind this is because Vitamin C stimulates the adrenal glands,[14] that produce among other things; collagen. Collagen is likened to a glue that holds the cells together. One of the first things I notice is that without enough Vitamin C, I start to develop hangnails. This is a sure sign that I need more.

Without enough collagen, a simple bump to the arm will cause these loosely bound cells to rupture, causing the blood to leak and pool under the skin as it does with bruises.

Without enough collagen high blood pressure can cause an artery to rupture and possibly lead to a stroke. There are other factors at play during a stroke, but Vitamin C certainly can minimize some of the surrounding circumstances.

Vitamin C is also well known for destroying several different kinds of bacteria and viruses,[15] as well as slowing the growth and effectiveness of any cells that may have survived.[16] Vitamin C is also non-specific,[17] so it will be effective on all kinds of bacteria and viruses no matter where they are in the body,[18] and how much they mutate from year to year. Tests also show that while small amounts of Vitamin C bring some immunity,[19] larger doses were even more effective.[20] One particular test showed that when Guinea pigs were injected with a bacterial infection, and then given large amounts of Vitamin C, 99 % of body cells showed bacterial destruction within the hour.[21] How's that for service?

There are countless studies that show how Vitamin C is extremely effective in improving the conditions of people with encephalitis, meningitis, poliomyelitis, pneumonia, tetanus/ lockjaw, and even very high fevers. While vaccines of today are not likely to give anyone the actual virus they are being vaccinated for, taking a nutritional supplement is certainly a simple and easy insurance policy to protect against that one in a million chance that it might. Large amounts of Vitamin C for an adult are considered to be 2-4 grams every 2-4 hours around the clock until symptoms subside. This would be way too much for a child or infant. Something as simple as a child gummy vitamin will go a long way to support their immunity but talk with your doctor before giving any supplement to anyone under 5 years of age.

When it comes to Vitamin C, the looming question is always how much is too much? Studies show that mammals that generate their own Vitamin C, consistently make it at about 35 milligrams per pound they weigh. That means a 175-pound man should be taking approximately 5 grams of Vitamin C a day. There are several factors that influence that, so it is not a fail-safe number, but it is a good place to start.

Vitamin C is also a detoxifier, so if someone lives in a semi-toxic environment, they might need a little more. Vitamin C is also burned up faster during times of stress, so that is another factor to consider when determining how much to take.

No matter how much you take, some is better than none, and more is better than some.[22] Each individual needs to find their own balance. I have heard a story about a Texas attorney who suffered from Phlebitis to the point that his doctor was considering amputation. He started taking as much as 25 grams of C per day, and the swelling started to go down immediately. Within 3 weeks, he was back to normal.

He continued to take this supplement until he was taking upwards of 40 grams per day. He then discovered his threshold. He developed a rash and had to reduce the amount until the rash went away. To each his own.

It is suggested that the average person between 100- 200 pounds, should take 500 to 1000 milligrams of Vitamin C if they are taking any kind of antibiotic or vaccination, twice a day for 3 days to help prevent any adverse reactions. If your child is smaller, talk with your doctor first and play it safe with 1-2 children's gummy vitamins per day, for a few days. A protein shake designed for kids is also a good choice. Young kids, and lighter weight individuals should not be treated like adults as their bodies are still learning how to adapt to the world around them.

For some people with any kind of intestinal swelling, such as Colitis or IBS, too much Vitamin C can sometimes cause diarrhea. This is because when the intestines are swollen, Vitamin C will reduce the swelling, and cause the intestinal tract to relax and begin releasing all the trapped bile stuck in between the folds. If this happens, simply reduce the amount of Vitamin C being taken, and make this transition more gradually.

B VITAMINS

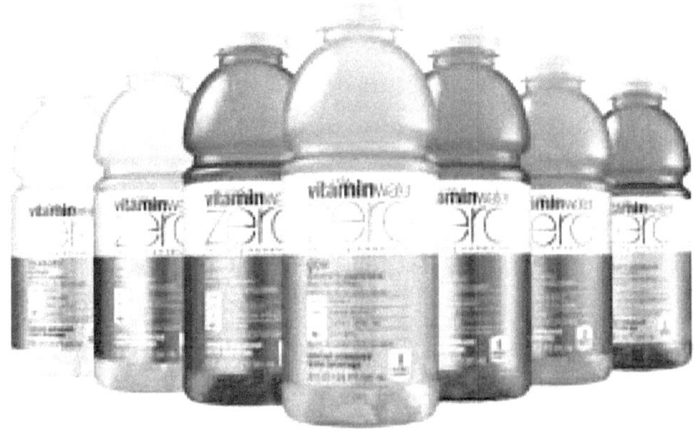

The B Vitamins also play a prominent role when fighting infections. To start with, Vitamin C is better utilized when taken along with Pantothenic Acid, also known as Vitamin B-5. This is particularly effective when combating the Polio virus. The B Vitamins are water soluble and not stored in the body, therefore they need to be eaten every day. We can't take too much as whatever is not used is simply lost in the urine.

The lymph glands produce antibodies and lymph cells that are needed to fight infections of all kinds. When these are swollen as with the Mumps, that means the Lymph system is at work. Animals deficient in Pantothenic Acid (Vitamin B-5) and Vitamin B-6 show a marked reduction in antibodies and White Blood Cells such that even after a vaccination, immunity is not increased.[23] So it makes sense that Pantothenic Acid / Vitamin B5 should be taken with any and all vaccines. Other studies show that there are some genetic families of rats that appear to need more Vitamin B-5 than others. Not only do they need more, but they are harmed more without it, much more than other rats from another genetic family.[24]

Further studies show that a low resistance to infection is a result of low Vitamin B-5[25] intake, more than any other nutrient.[26] Without Vitamin B-5, vaccines for sore throat, pharyngitis, tetanus, typhoid, and polio, showed no increased immunity, because *vaccines don't increase white blood cells, they only stimulate them.*[27] It is vital to increase white cell count, before the body can effectively stimulate them. As little as 40 mg of Vitamin B-6 will increase white blood cell counts and antibody production within 3 hours.[28]

It is best to take a B-complex supplement where you can get all the B- Vitamins at once, since they complement each other. Taking just one of them can cause an imbalance. Taking them on an empty stomach can also cause some nausea so taking them with a little protein such as some banana, or a glass of milk, with help to take them easily without any negative effects. I prefer some brand of Vitamin Water because I can drink them all day and get hydrated at the same time. All the B Vitamins are needed, but of them all, Vitamin B-5 played the biggest role in fighting infections.

VITAMIN A

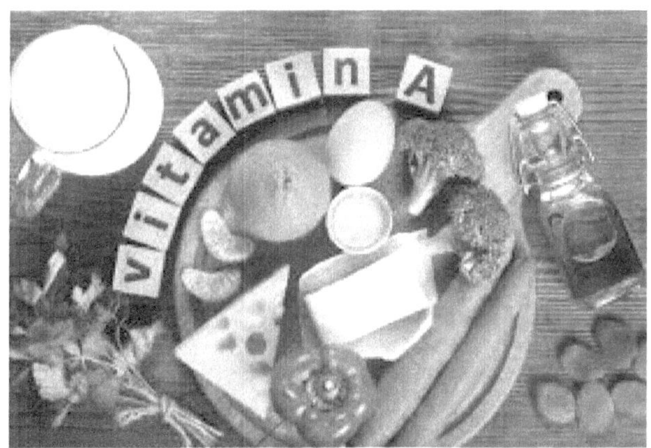

Vitamin A is another supplement that is used up quickly during and infectious period,[29] particularly during a bout with Measles and a high fever.[30] It is usually spilled out in the urine[31] when the body comes under stress of any kind. Without an adequate amount of Vitamin A, millions of dead cells fall onto the mucous membrane linings within the body cavities. Here, they begin to collect and provide an abundant supply of food for the invading bacteria and virus.

When there is enough Vitamin A, these membranes are routinely washed clean and become more efficient at both producing white blood cells,[32] and at transporting them throughout the body.[33]

When enough Vitamin A is present it also helps to prevent infections of the skin, and eyes, and especially the cornea within the eyes, places that are not easily reached except from within.

Cortisone shots are known to increase the need for Vitamin A[34] as well as other nutrients because they are a form of stress, particularly during bouts with rheumatic fever, encephalitis, measles, and streptococcus.

Even if someone has already fallen into the grip of one of these diseases, Vitamin A has been known to shorten the duration of measles, scarlet fever, pneumonia, infections of the eyes, middle ear, sinuses, kidneys, intestines, ovaries, and uterus[35], and promote a quicker recovery. Along with Vitamin C, Vitamin A is one of the first supplements that should be taken orally. An average appropriate amount would be approximately 25,000 units per day until the infection subsides, and then reducing the mounts to 15,000 units per day to maintain. Because Vitamin A is stored in the tissues and primarily the liver, it is possible to get too much, however, as much as 200,000 units a day has

been given by doctors for up to six months[36]
without any toxicity, the risk of toxicity is very low.
When we consider all the good that Vitamin A does,
it is better to keep your levels high. It is suggested
that 25,000 units daily is a safe and effective
amount.[37]

Vitamin A can also be applied topically, and has
been known to be very effective against impetigo,
boils, carbuncles, and open ulcers, particularly
when applied locally.[38] There are two basic topical
ointments on the market, one oil based, and one
water based. They will both work well, however I
prefer water based as I believe it can be absorbed
faster. One of the concerns in taking Vitamin A is
that it can be damaged by Oxygen, [39] for this
reason, a Vitamin E supplement would be another
helpful supplement to take during times of stress
and infection.

VITAMIN E

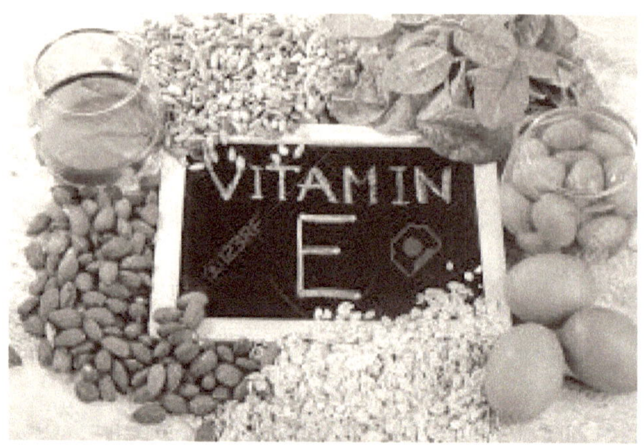

Vitamin E serves many purposes in the everyday work of the human body, mainly serving as an anti-oxidant against both organs and tissues. One of the other important features is to diminish and even replace scar tissue. Any high fever can potentially cause scar tissue, especially during Rheumatic Fever, Nephritis, and Measles. Measles have been known to cause scar tissue in the eyes damaging them permanently.

There are actually eight forms of Vitamin E when it is derived from its natural state. Alpha-, Bata-, Gamma-, and Delta-tocopherol; as well as Alph-, Beta-, Gama-, Delta-tocotrienol. When taken as one surce of Vitamin E, they are nontoxic and far more potent. What we buy in the store is only one of the eight, Alpha-tocopherol. Like Vitamin C, some is better than none, so the choice is really about how much effort you choose to put into your recovery. As always, I always advocate eating the natural food before supplements, but statistics show that more people rarely eat enough unprocessed food as ready-to-eat meals are so much easier to prepare.

PROTEIN

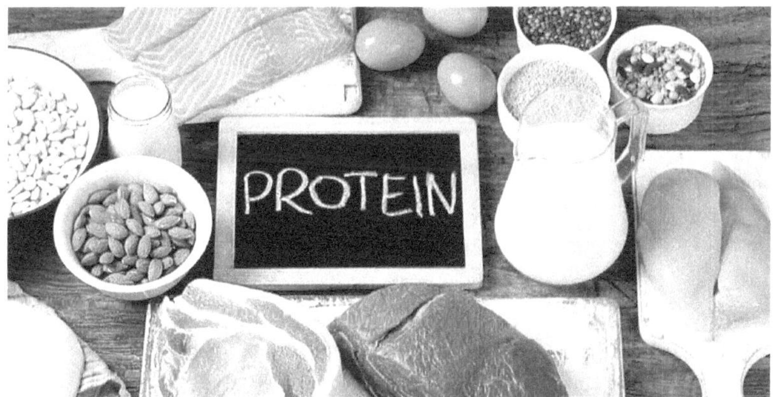

Protein supplements are another one of those vital supplements that most people take for granted. You don't have to be a weightlifter to require more protein in the average diet. Antibodies, white blood cells, lymph cells are all made of protein, and without enough protein, Vitamin C has a fraction of its effectiveness.

When low protein diets are replaced with higher protein diets, the production of antibodies increases a hundred-fold within a few hours. Some of the best sources of this protein include Liver, Yeast, and especially Wheat Germ.[40] Eggs, Meat, Milk, and Soy are also great sources of the kind of protein that raises White Blood Cell counts.[41] In all cases, whenever the nutrition is improved, whether through natural food, or supplements, an increase in all of the bodies defense mechanisms will increases in function and performance.[42]

ACIDOSIS

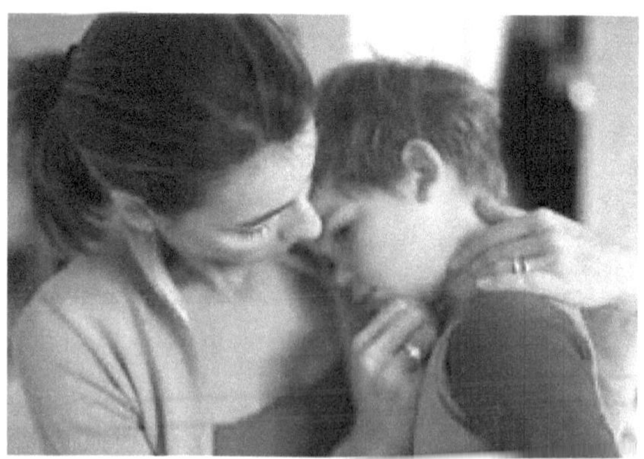

Feeling nauseous during any illness can be a real threat when someone is already sick. Feeling sick can interfere with getting the real nutrition we need at a time like this. Dehydration will happen quickly when someone is losing body fluids through diarrhea and vomiting.

To quell the nausea, try taking a small amount of natural sugars such as orange juice, a teaspoon of honey, or applesauce. By ingesting these sugars at the beginning of the sickness, and taking them every hour or two, you will get to the point where you can start rehydrating, and then on to eating solid food again.

Start with a vitamin supplemented water to replace the B Vitamins, and to get a jump start on recovery. After getting back to the point where you are able to eat again, start slowly with small amounts of fruit and broths. Bananas are always a good place to start because they are soft, full of protein and nutrition.

Once you are ready to start eating again, add the supplements slowly and don't be in a big hurry to get back to work. We typically get sick because we didn't take the time to get some rest and eat right in the first place.

By taking vaccinations as they are needed, they are not dangerous, and they don't give people disease. When taken properly, and adding some added nutrition, vaccinations provide an additional level of protection from all the very dangerous diseases surrounding all of us every day.

Between the nutrition and the vaccinations, there is no reason any reasonably healthy person can't go forward without any concerns of contracting some debilitating disease as we walk through life.

Nutritional Therapy's Medical Disclaimer

The information on this site is not intended to be a substitute for professional medical advice, diagnosis or treatment. Each individual person has their own unique set of medical needs, and all information gathered here should be considered along with the advice of the reader's doctor. This information is intended to offer as a supplement to traditional, drug related medical therapies, and the readers assume all responsibility when putting this information into effect. This information is accurate and true to the best of all authors' authority; is taken from numerous medical sources and referenced whenever possible. All content, including text, graphics, images and information, contained on or available through this publication is for general information purposes and does not take into account any other preexisting conditions. Readers will not hold NUTRITIONAL THERAPY'S authors or administrators responsible for any adverse results.

NEVER DISREGARD PROFESSIONAL MEDICAL TREATMENT BECAUSE OF SOMETHING YOU HAVE READ ON OR ACCESSED THROUGH THIS MATERIAL.

Nutritional-Therapy will not be responsible or liable for any course of treatment, diagnosis, or any other information, services or products that are obtained through this publication; but they offer alternatives to those wanting to get away from prescription drugs; and those wanting to restore health naturally without them.

For more information, please contact NutritionalTherapyUS@gmail.com

You are encouraged to report negative side effects of prescription drugs to the FDA. Visit the FDA MedWatch website; http://www.fda.gov/Safety/MedWatch/HowToReport/default.htm or call 1-800-FDA-1088 to find out more.

To find out more about Nutritional Therapy, and author Kerri Ryan, go to

www.Nutritional-Therapy.us

www.Amazon.com/author/kerriryan

Endnotes

1 https://www.cdc.gov/vaccinesafety/concerns/index.html

2 [46]

3 [47]

4 [48] -

5 https://vaccines.procon.org/

6

7 https://www.cdc.gov/vaccines/parents/diseases/diseases-forgot.html?CDC_AA_refVal=https%3A%2F%2Fwww.cdc.gov%2Fvaccines%2Fparents%2Fdiseases%2Fchild%2F14-diseases.html

8Banerjee, S. et al., J. of Bio. Chem. 190,177, 1951; Stefanini, M., et al, Proc. Soc. Ewp. Bio. Med. 75, 806, 1950

9 Banerjee, S. et al., J. of Bio. Chem. 190,177, 1951, Stefanini, M., et al, Proc. Soc. Ewp. Bio. Med. 75, 806, 1950

10 Cuttle, T.D., Quart. J., Med. 7,575, 1938; Neander, G., Acta Med.. Scand. 109,453, 1942

11 Nungester, W.J., et al, J. Infect. Dis., 83, 50, 1948; Faulkner, J.M, New England J. Med., 213, 19, 1935

12 Faulkner, J.M, New England J. Med., 213, 19, 1935; Crandon, J.H., et al, New England J. Med. 223, 353, 1940;

13 Stefanini, M., et al, Proc. Soc. Ewp. Bio. Med. 75, 806, 1950

14 Banerjee, S. et al., J. of Bio. Chem. 190,177, 1951, Stefanini, M., et al, Proc. Soc. Ewp. Bio. Med. 75, 806, 1950

15 Kligler, I.J., et al, J. Path. Bact. 46, 619, 1938; Jungblut, C.W., J. Exp. Med. 70, 315.1939

16 Kligler, I.J., et al, J. Path. Bact. 46, 619, 1938; Jungblut, C.W., J. Exp. Med. 33, 203.1937; Jungblut, C.W., J. Exp. Med. 70, 315.1939

17 Klenner, F.R., TriState Med. J. July 1954; Klenner, F.R., TriState Med. J. Sept 1956; Klenner, F.R., TriState Med. J. June 1957; Klenner, F.R., TriState Med. J. Feb. 1960

18 Kligler, I.J., et al, J. Path. Bact. 46, 619, 1938, Knight, C.A. et al, J. Exp, Med. 79,29, 1944

19 Burkhaug, K. E., Acta Tubercul. Scand. Scand., 1939; ,Steinbach, M.M., et al, Am. Rev. Tubercul. 43, 401, 414, 1941

20 Burkhaug, K. E., Acta Tubercul. Scand. Scand., 1939- Steinbach, M.M., et al, Am. Rev. Tubercul. 43, 401, 414, 1941

21 Burkhaug, K. E., Acta Tubercul. Scand. Scand., 1939- Steinbach, M.M., et al, Am. Rev. Tubercul. 43, 401, 414, 1941

22 Burkhaug, K. E., Acta Tubercul. Scand. Scand., 1939- Steinbach, M.M., et al, Am. Rev. Tubercul. 43, 401, 414, 1941

23 Clark, I., et al, Endocrinology 56, 232, 1955; Ludovici, P.P., et al, Proc. Soc. Wxp. Biol. Med. 77, 526, 1951; Alexrod, A.E., Nut. Rev. 10, 353, 1952; Alexrod, A.E. et al, Ann. N.Y., Acad, Sci. Acad, Sci. 63, 202. 1955; Axelrod, A.E., J. Nut. 72, 325, 1960;

24 Williams, R.J., Biochemical Individuality, Wiley, NY, NY, 1956; Seronde, J., et al, J. Inf. Dis., 97,35, 1955

25 Seronde, J., et al, J. Inf. Dis., 97,35, 1955

26 Clark, I., et al, Endocrinology 56, 232, 1955

27 Clark, I., et al, Endocrinology 56, 232, 1955; Ludovici, P.P., et al, Proc. Soc. Wxp. Biol. Med. 77, 526, 1951; Alexrod, A.E., Nut. Rev. 10, 353, 1952; Alexrod, A.E. et al, Ann. N.Y., Acad, Sci. Acad, Sci. 63, 202. 1955; Axelrod, A.E., J. Nut. 72, 325, 1960;

28 Yamada, K., et al, J. Vitaminol, 5, 188, 1959

29 Spector, S., et al, Am. J. Dis. Child. 66, 376, 1943; Brenner, S., et al, Arch. Int. Med. 71, 482, 1943; Popper, H., et al, Proc. Soc. Exp. Biol. Med. 68, 676, 1948

30 Josephs, H.W., Am. J. Dis. Child. 65, 712, 1943

31 Jacobs, A.L., et al, J. Clin. Nut. 2,155, 1954

32 Ludovici, P.P., et al, Proc. Soc. Wxp. Biol. Med. 77, 526, 1951; Alexrod, A.E., Nut. Rev. 10, 353, 1952; Alexrod, A.E. et al, Ann. N.Y., Acad, Sci. Acad, Sci. 63, 202. 1955

33 Wolf, J., Nut. Rev.20, 161, 1962

34 Clark, I., et al, Endocrinology 56, 232, 1955

35 Green, H.N., et al, Brit. Med. J. 2, 595, 1931;Kahn, R.H., Am. J. Anatomy, 95, 309, 1954

36 Pinkerton, H., et al, Science 89, 368, 1939, Porter, A.D., et al, Brit, J. Derm. 62, 355, 1950

37 Abbott, O.D., et al, Am. J. Physiology 126, 254, 1939 Porter, A.D., et al, Brit, J. Derm. 62, 355, 1950

38 Yamada, K., et al, J. Vitaminol, 5, 188, 1959; Porter, A.D., et al, Brit, J. Derm. 62, 355, 1950; Porter, A.D., Brit. J. Derm. 63, 123, 1951; Jacobs, A.L., et al, J. Clin. Nut. 2, 155, 1954

39 Moore, T, Biochem. J. 34, 1321, 1940

40 Ershoff, B,H., Nut, 13, 33, 1955; O'Dell, B.L., et al, Arch. Biochem. Biophysics, 54, 232, 1955

41 Guggenheim, K., et al, J. Immunol. 58, 133, 1948

42 Guggenheim, K., et al, J. Immunol. 58, 133, 1948

There is a common misconception that by taking vaccinations, one can actually contract the disease. The truth is immunizations are made from a weakened pathogen, that is incapable of transmitting the disease. The problems that can come up come not from the vaccine, but from the recipient's inability to protect themselves from it. By adding a few simple nutritional supplements, you can prime the body to receive a new pathogen, and successfully activate the benefits they bring.

On the other hand, by refusing to take vaccinations, you will be putting yourself and your children in harm's way and risking almost certain infection. Learn the Truth, take the proper action, and go on to live a happy, healthy life.

9 781703 282795